MAKE YOUR OWN HAND SANITIZER

How to Make Your Own Hand Sanitizer with Ingredients You Always Have at Home

© **Copyright 2020 by Mark Fine**

All rights reserved.

This document is geared towards providing exact and reliable information with regards to the topic and issue covered. The publication is sold with the idea that the publisher is not required to render accounting, officially permitted, or otherwise, qualified services. If advice is necessary, legal or professional, a practiced individual in the profession should be ordered.

- From a Declaration of Principles which was accepted and approved equally by a Committee of the American Bar Association and a Committee of Publishers and Associations.

In no way is it legal to reproduce, duplicate, or transmit any part of this document in either electronic means or in printed format. Recording of this publication is strictly prohibited and any storage of this document is not allowed unless with written permission from the publisher. All rights reserved.

The information provided herein is stated to be truthful and consistent, in that any liability, in terms of inattention or otherwise, by any usage or abuse of any policies, processes, or directions contained within is the solitary and utter responsibility of the recipient reader. Under no circumstances will any legal responsibility or blame be held against the publisher for any reparation, damages, or monetary loss due to the information herein, either directly or indirectly.

Respective authors own all copyrights not held by the publisher.

The information herein is offered for informational purposes solely, and is universal as so. The presentation of the information is without contract or any type of guarantee assurance.

The trademarks that are used are without any consent, and the publication of the trademark is without permission or backing by the trademark owner. All trademarks and brands within this book are for clarifying purposes only and are the owned by the owners themselves, not affiliated with this document

TABLE OF CONTENTS

Introduction 1

Chapter one: Make your own hand sanitizer 5

Chapter two: How washing your hands keeps
you healthy 28

Chapter three: Why you should wash your hands 37

Chapter four: Can you drink hand sanitizer
or get drunk on it 52

Chapter five: Health and hand sanitation 63

Chapter six: How does hand sanitizer work 72

Conclusion 82

INTRODUCTION

There are many myths and misconceptions about hand sanitizers. In this eBook, we're going to look at some facts to debunk the myths and set the record straight. One of the most popular misconceptions is that hand sanitizers are virtually infallible and that they can prevent the spread of all contagious diseases, including the cold or flu. Although a hand sanitizer can kill more than 60 percent of flu viruses on your hand, most people actually contract flu from airborne agents, by breathing in the germs.

So even if you've used a sanitizing product, and your hands are clean and germ-free, you can still catch or spread the virus. A hand sanitizer may actually be a more potent preventive mechanism for gastrointestinal diseases, rather than infections such as the cold or flu.

Another myth is that they are not as effective as conventional hand-washing with soap and water, in eliminating germs from hands. This is not necessarily true. Washing with soap and water works betters if your hands are visibly soiled, that is if you have dirt in your hands. However, if your hands look clean but are actually ridden with germs, then an alcohol-based hand sanitizer is a better option because the alcohol is more effective in killing the germs.

Another myth is that hand sanitizer's lead to dry hands. These products contain emollients, which are chemicals that reduce irritation by protecting and soothing the skin. As counterintuitive as it may seem, an alcohol-based hand sanitizer is actually less harsh on the skin than soap and water. A study conducted by Brown University researchers found that washing your hands with soap and water leads to skin that may look and feel quite dry. A hand sanitizer, on the other hand, may keep hands moisturized.

You can make a somewhat effective sanitizer at home. While homemade variants may be cheaper, most don't contain the recommended 60 percent alcohol content, which experts agree is the optimum concentration to eliminate germs. Understandably, the best results are seen with brand names, such as Purell or Germ X.

However, as long as the product contains 60 percent alcohol, a generic brand will work just as fine as a premium store brand. You don't have to pay the higher price for a brand name product.

Compiling all the hand sanitizer facts, we can safely say that an alcohol-based sanitizer is the most effective means to kill germs in our hands, but only as long as the product is used sparingly and responsibly.

An alcohol-based sanitizer is not only able to eliminate more germs than soap and water, but it is also gentler on the skin if used in moderate amounts. And when supervised by an adult, this product can be safe for kids as well.

While alcohol-based sanitizers have faced criticism of late, mainly due to the high alcohol concentration, experts say that some of these fears are unfounded. Alcohol is not absorbed into the skin to any degree to warrant these fears. Even with excessive usage, the level of alcohol absorption is harmless at best. Alcohol may contribute to some sanitizer dangers, but not to any great extent.

The argument against alcohol content only holds up if the products are used in a way that they were not intended to be used in. For example, an alcohol-based hand sanitizer is not meant to be ingested, but there have been several cases where children, as well as adults, have consumed the liquid and fallen very ill.

Some manufacturers have attempted to address the public's concern over alcohol content and started making alcohol free variants as a safer alternative. These products rely on plant oils to neutralize germs, but so far have not been as effective as alcohol-based hand sanitizers. If used properly, an alcohol-based hand sanitizer is no more dangerous than an alcohol-free variant.

CHAPTER ONE

MAKE YOUR OWN HAND SANITIZER

Some business hand sanitizer contains ingredients as terrifying as the germs they shield you from, so why not make your own hand sanitizer from fixings you select? This is a superb task for kids just as grown-ups since the venture can be extended to incorporate a conversation about cleanliness and sterilization. You'll set aside cash, shield yourself from germs, and can tweak the aroma of the hand sanitizer so it doesn't smell restorative.

Hand cleanliness is one of the essential techniques used to decrease the fecal-oral transmission of irresistible operators. In any case, clashing hand cleanliness proposals for various settings are creating turmoil among the overall population concerning what is the best practice to follow or what items ought to be utilized for everyday handwashing and hand cleanliness. This record gives the data important to average purchasers to settle on an educated choice.

Understanding Your Immediate Environment Many individuals have the confusion that their quick condition must be without germ. Notwithstanding, this is just conceivable in a genuine sans germ chamber in a lab or in certain clinic settings. We live in a characteristic world that is brimming with microorganisms, living things that can't be seen by our exposed eyes. While a portion of the microorganisms can cause ailment or ailments, others can be fundamental to our condition and prosperity. Albeit a few microorganisms can cause nourishment decay or infections, a considerable lot of them is a characteristic piece of our food sources and situations.

Without great microscopic organisms, you would be without your preferred yogurt, sauerkraut, or certain drugs! Bovines would not have the option to utilize grasses for vitality without great microbial accomplices. What's more, without acceptable microbes or growths, our earth would be loaded with yard squander and other natural rubbish. Moreover, we ought not to overlook that our typical, solid body has different outside boundaries and inner components (safe framework) to battle germs, as long as their numbers are not overpowering.

In this way, comprehension and figuring out how to control or manage both the great and the awful microorganisms on our body and in our condition can assist us with utilizing those organisms, and simultaneously, limit the spread of transmittable illnesses. The objective is to decrease the number of awful microorganisms to a level low enough for the body to sensibly fend them off with its current resistant framework.

The Body's Bugs

The body portions of solid people and creatures are hosts to an assortment of organisms known as inhabitant microorganisms. Be that as it may, through contact with different articles, the body likewise gets different microorganisms known as transient organisms. For instance, a normal individual's hand can convey 10,000 to 10 million microscopic organisms, some occupant and some transient. At the point when people or creatures are wiped out or tainted with explicit organisms, the quantity of microorganisms may increment.

The skin isn't the main host territory on our bodies for microorganisms and different organisms. Numerous organisms are likewise present in the intestinal tracts of people and creatures. These are known as fecal microorganisms. An individual's hands, arms, or fingers may get sullied with fecal microorganisms in the wake of utilizing the latrine.

These must be evacuated by the mechanical grinding of washing with cleanser and water or devastated by the utilization of disinfectant arrangements. The microorganisms from human and creature sources can be transmitted to hands, others, nourishments, and whatever else that the hand interacts with and the other way around. This is the reason acceptable handwashing is significant for decreasing hurtful microorganisms on all fours lessening the danger of moving destructive microorganisms to other people.

How It Works

The dynamic fixing right now the recipe is the alcohol, which needs to include in any event 60% of the item so as to be a successful disinfectant. The formula calls for 99% isopropyl alcohol (scouring alcohol) or ethanol (grain alcohol, most normally accessible at 90%-95%). Kindly don't utilize some other sorts of alcohol (e.g., methanol, butanol), as they are lethal. Additionally, on the off chance that you utilize an item that contains a lower level of alcohol (e.g., 70% alcohol) at that point you have to expand the measure of alcohol in the formula or it won't be as viable.

Fundamental Oils in Hand Sanitizer

Notwithstanding adding scent to your hand sanitizer, the fundamental oil you pick may likewise help ensure you against germs. For instance, thyme and clove oil have antimicrobial properties. In the event that you are utilizing antimicrobial oils, just utilize a drop or two, since these oils will, in general, be extremely groundbreaking and may bother your skin. Different oils, for example, lavender or chamomile, may help relieve your skin. Tea tree oil is antimicrobial. Two or three drops might be added to the formula, yet it's imperative to note numerous individuals are touchy to this oil, in any event, when it's weakened.

What You'll Need

Hardware/Tools

- Bowl and spoon
- Funnel
- Bottle with siphon distributor

Materials

- 2/3 cup 99 percent scouring alcohol (isopropyl alcohol) or ethanol
- 1/3 cup aloe vera gel
- 8 to 10 drops basic oil, discretionary

Steps to Make It

Make Hand Sanitizer

Nothing could be simpler! Essentially combine the fixings and afterward utilize the pipe to empty them into the jug. Screw the siphon back onto the container and you're all set.

- Gather Your Ingredients

Ensure you have your scouring alcohol, aloe vera gel, and discretionary basic oils prepared and allotted.

Blend Ingredients

Include all fixings together in your bowl and blend completely with a spoon.

Immerse Your Bottle

Utilizing the channel, cautiously empty your DIY hand sanitizer into your preferred jug, screw the highest point of your jug on tight, and start utilizing.

Substitutions

The key fixing close by sanitizer is alcohol, so it's conceivable to fill in for the aloe vera gel. The motivation behind the aloe gel is to ensure hands against the drying impacts of alcohol. Fundamentally, it's a humectant. This implies it helps lock in dampness. Different humectants which could be utilized instead of aloe incorporate glycerin or hand salve. Be that as it may, it's as yet critical to keep the alcohol in the last item in any event 60%. In the event that you can't discover alcohol, the best alternative is to wash your hands with cleanser and water as opposed to endeavor a custom made hand sanitizer formula.

Working with 70% Alcohol

Scouring alcohol and ethanol from a store will, in

general, be either 90-99% alcohol or, more than likely 70% alcohol. You can sterilize your hands with 70% alcohol, yet there does next to no you can add to it (possibly a couple of drops of fundamental oil or jojoba oil, to improve fragrance or surface). Blending 70% alcohol in with different fixings weakens the alcohol, so it's anything but difficult to dip under the 60% alcohol prescribed by the CDC.

Ensure Your Hands

Alcohol dries the skin and strips defensive oils. Follow up a hand sanitizer (or handwashing) with a decent cream to keep skin fit as a fiddle. Harmed skin has little splits that trap microscopic organisms and infections and make them harder to evacuate. In the event that you have delicate skin, attempt to keep the measure of alcohol close by sanitizer around 60-70% (as right now) a higher focus may cause bothering.

DIY Hand Sanitizer Gel Recipe

Here's the way to make your own one of a kind DIY hand sanitizer.

- 2 parts Rubbing Alcohol (at any rate 90%, yet

ideally 99%)

- 1 part Aloe Vera Gel (the less added substances the better)

- 10 drops Essential Oils (discretionary - consider ones that have extra germicide properties, for example, lavender, thyme, clove, cinnamon leaf, peppermint and so on.)

- Plastic squirt container or siphon

The most effective method to Make Hand Sanitizer

Consolidate all fixings together, mix well, and fill a press bottle (with a channel). Done! You have to utilize at least 60% scouring alcohol for this to be a compelling germ warrior so beginning within any event 90% scouring alcohol (not 70%), is an unquestionable requirement. You can discover scouring alcohol as high as 99% which will be significantly increasingly viable. Likewise - be cautioned: basic oils that are known to have against microbial properties can be a skin aggravation to those with touchy skin. Utilize fewer drops, or join with alleviating oils for an increasingly adjusted formula (for example camomile). This saves for around a half year.

Results

It works! It smelled solid however the smell dispersed truly quickly and my hands weren't withered old witch hands in the wake of utilizing it. I wonder if this would work utilizing plain shea margarine however I don't think enough about science to decide whether that would be a steady blend (see, I don't simply make things up or enlighten you concerning things I think will work). A few people include a tablespoon of vegetable glycerine to the aloe vera for extra dampness. I may attempt this with the following bunch.

Triclosan

Alright, you have my consideration. I'm the greatest recuperating depressed person you'll ever meet and this is a trendy expression for me. In any case, I've learned through my common examinations to look into trustworthy sources before closing anything (and to not check Web MD continually either). With the goal that's what I did when I saw this hot little word. As indicated by the FDA site (I hear these folks comprehend what they are discussing, just sayin'):

Different investigations in microorganisms have raised the likelihood that triclosan adds to making microbes impervious to anti-toxins. FDA doesn't have adequate wellbeing proof to prescribe changing customer utilization of items that contain triclosan as of now. Right now, FDA doesn't have proof that triclosan added to antibacterial cleansers and body washes gives additional medical advantages over cleanser and water. Shoppers worried about utilizing hand and body cleansers with triclosan should wash with customary cleanser and water

So on one hand, Triclosan could be a known supporter of making protection from anti-microbials however then again, there is no strong evidence that it works any superior to cleanser or water. I have sensitivities to two or three anti-infection agents as of now, so for me, I feel it bodes well to avoid Triclosan. That doesn't mean everybody needs to, you simply need to settle on an educated choice.

Alcohol Free Hand Sanitizer Gel

- 1 cup unadulterated aloe vera gel
- 1-2 teaspoons of witch hazel (include until the ideal consistency is come to)
- 8 drops of basic oils

Generally Alcohol-Free Hand Sanitizer Gel

- 2 cups unadulterated aloe vera gel
- 2 tablespoons 90% SD40 alcohol (perfumer's alcohol on the off chance that you can get it)
- 2-3 teaspoons basic oils

Alcohol based Hand Sanitizer

- 1/4 cup unadulterated aloe vera gel
- 1/4 cup grain alcohol or vodka
- 10 drops basic oils

Tiffany Muehlbauer has been discovering her way back to an increasingly maintainable way of life throughout the previous quite a while. During that venture, she has rediscovered a significant number of the home cures and homegrown plans that our predecessors utilized, yet that such a large number of us have ever been told or overlooked throughout the years. The expansion of a little girl to her family about a year prior has significantly expanded her longing to live more naturally and to free her life of unneeded and undesirable synthetic concoctions.

Today, sanitizers are utilized for something other than limited-time giveaways. More organizations, from Fortune 500 organizations to schools and daycare focuses, are buying them to help lessen non-attendance. The Advertising Specialty Institute (ASI), one of the business' biggest exchange associations, has declared that hand sanitizers presently rival pens as one of the most mainstream logo things for promoting. Brilliant organizations are parting with them to customers and workers the same.

Furthermore, the Center for Disease Control and Prevention (CDC) recommends that when cleanser and water are not accessible, alcohol based dispensable hand wipes, splashes, or gels sanitizers might be utilized to help forestall the spread of germs.

Hand sanitizer sprays have become extremely well known on the grounds that they are little, modest and helpfully conveyed in a pocket or satchel anyplace. As a public expo giveaway, limited time hand sanitizers are a successful and helpful item, yet satisfying to the corporate spending plan. The introduction these items can give an organization brand is definitely justified even despite the low expenses and elevates a positive attitude to any individual who gets one. A couple of the choices for kinds of sanitizers, which can all be marked with your organization name or logo, include:

- Sprays
- Sanitizer Gels
- Soaps
- Wipes

Because of the expanding prominence of hand sanitizers, a wide range of bundling alternatives has been presented. A few models incorporate antibacterial smaller than usual, miniaturized scale, and carefully designed sprayers. There are other pressing choices accessible also, for example, official pocket sprayers, antibacterial charge cards, and lighter molded sprayers. What's more, you would now be able to purchase pocket siphons just as pocket siphon and sprayer units.

Other than pocket-size things, there are likewise antibacterial moist disposable cloth canisters and pockets, froth cleansers, sanitizer wipe parcels, and moist disposable cloth units. A portion of the fresher alternatives incorporate carabiner bested bottles, turn-lock sprayers, official style sprayers, and sanitizers with carabiners, chains, or key rulers connected. These are extraordinary for a helpful yet without hands choice that is anything but difficult to snatch.

Insightful organizations, schools and different gatherings today are joining the numerous mindful people that are having any kind of effect by assisting with controlling the spread of infections with limited time hand sanitizers. Altered with your image before the influenza season hits these can help decrease truancy busy working and school. If that wasn't already enough with a logo or topic engraved on the item the business will increase rehashed presentation for their image again and again.

Is it safe?

DIY hand sanitizer plans are everywhere throughout the web nowadays - yet would they say they are protected?

These plans, including the ones above, are proposed for use by experts with both the skill and assets to securely make custom made hand sanitizers. Custom made hand sanitizer is possibly prescribed in extraordinary circumstances when you can't wash your hands for years to come.

I will-advised fixings or extents can prompt:

- lack of adequacy, implying that the sanitizer may not successfully take out the danger of introduction to a few or all microorganisms
- skin disturbance, injury, or consumes
- exposure to dangerous synthetic concoctions by means of inward breath

Custom made hand sanitizer is additionally not suggested for use with youngsters. Youngsters might be progressively inclined to ill-advised hand sanitizer utilization, which could prompt more serious hazards for injury.

The most effective method to utilize hand sanitizer

Two things to know about when utilizing hand sanitizer is that you have to rub it into your skin until your hands are dry. Also, if your hands are oily or grimy, you should wash them first with cleanser and water.

In light of that, here are a few hints for utilizing hand sanitizer successfully.

- Spray or apply the sanitizer to the palm of one hand.
- Thoroughly rub your hands together. Ensure you spread the whole surface of your hands and every one of your fingers.
- Continue scouring for 30 to 60 seconds or until your hands are dry. It can take at any rate 60 seconds and at times longer, for hand sanitizer to kill most germs.

What germs can hand sanitizer murder?

As indicated by the CDCTrusted Source, a alcohol

based hand sanitizer that meets the alcohol volume prerequisite can rapidly decrease the number of organisms on your hands. It can likewise help obliterate a wide scope of malady causing operators or pathogens on your hands, including the novel coronavirus SARS-CoV-2.

Be that as it may, even the best alcohol based hand sanitizers have restrictions and don't take out a wide range of germs.

As indicated by the CDC, hand sanitizers won't dispose of possibly unsafe synthetics. It's likewise not viable at slaughtering the accompanying germs:

- norovirus
- cryptosporidium (which causes cryptosporidiosis)
- clostridium difficile (otherwise called C. diff)

Additionally, a hand sanitizer may not function admirably if your hands are unmistakably filthy or oily. This may occur in the wake of working with nourishment, accomplishing yard work, cultivating, or playing a game.

On the off chance that your hands look grimy or vile, decide on handwashing rather than a hand sanitizer.

Handwashing versus hand sanitizer

Realizing when it's ideal to wash your hands, and when hand sanitizers can be useful, it is vital to shield yourself from the novel coronavirus just as different sicknesses, similar to the regular cold and occasional influenza.

While both fill a need, washing your hands with cleanser and water ought to consistently be a need, as indicated by the CDC. Possibly use hand sanitizer on the off chance that your cleanser and water isn't accessible in a given circumstance.

It's likewise critical to consistently wash your hands:

- after setting off to the washroom
- after cleaning out your nose, hacking, or wheezing
- before eating
- after contacting surfaces that could be debased

The CDC records explicit instructions-Trusted

Source on the best method to wash your hands. This is the thing that they suggest:

- Always utilize spotless, running water. (It very well may be warm or cold.)
- Wet your hands first, at that point turn the water off, and foam your hands with cleanser.
- Rub your hands together with the cleanser for in any event 20 seconds. Make a point to clean the rear of your hands, between your fingers and under your nails.
- Turn the water on and wash your hands. Utilize a spotless towel or air dry.

Hand sanitizer is convenient in a hurried approach to help forestall the spread of germs when cleanser and water isn't accessible. Alcohol based hand sanitizers can help keep you safe and lessen the spread of the novel coronavirus.

On the off chance that you are making some hard memories discovering hand sanitizer at your neighborhood stores and handwashing isn't accessible, you can find a way to make your own. You just need a couple of fixings, for example, scouring alcohol, aloe vera gel, and a basic oil or lemon juice.

In spite of the fact that hand sanitizers can be a compelling method for disposing of germs, wellbeing specialists despite everything prescribe handwashing at whatever point conceivable to keep your hands liberated from infection-causing infections and different germs.

Is Germ X Hand Sanitizer Effective, and If So, Why?

Here are a couple of realities that should respond to the inquiry 'Is Germ X hand sanitizer compelling?'

Hand sanitizer when all is said in done slaughters, in any event, the same number of germs as cleanser and water. It has been known for a long time that washing your hands consistently keeps one from getting a wide range of disorders and assists with keeping you solid generally speaking. Most hand sanitizers murder almost 100% of all germs on your hands when you use them.

Hand sanitizers are not costly and along these lines, there is actually no rhyme or reason why you ought not to utilize them, particularly on the off chance that you have at least one youngsters. Children will in general touch a wide range of grimy things over the span of the day; truth be told, some appear to try contacting however many filthy things as could be allowed and afterward placing their fingers in their eyes, mouth or up their nose. Having something directly close by to clean their hands will forestall they're becoming ill and that, however, instruct them great wellbeing propensities at an early age.

Germ X sanitizers specifically are powerful as well as simple to utilize. You can get moist disposable clothes that are anything but difficult to use on infants and little youngsters, froth sanitizers that are kid cordial and sanitizers that have nutrient E included. There are likewise Germ X sanitizers that have unique aromas included, from aloe to tangerine to lavender.

It's anything but a specific brand that is compelling however the way that keeping the hands clean is a certain fire approach to remain sound and forestall infection and ailment. There are additionally some specific hand sanitizers available that you might need to consider, for example, ones that battle MRSA. MRSA executes a large number of individuals consistently and gets into the circulatory system by means of cuts and open injuries. While specific enemy of MRSA hand sanitizer is somewhat pricier than normal sanitizer, it very well may be a smart thought to keep this in your home's medical aid unit. You can get either the wipe variant or the froth adaptation of the sanitizer and use it on the off chance that you or one of your children gets a cut.

On the off chance that you are not particularly specific about what sort of sanitizer you need, at that point it is sufficiently simple to purchase any sort at a market or store. The cost fluctuates relying upon the specific kind and brand name you purchase yet, as a rule, they are modest and definitely justified even despite the cost.

CHAPTER TWO
HOW WASHING YOUR HANDS KEEPS YOU HEALTHY

Contact is one of the manners in which individuals connect with their general surroundings. If you attempted to monitor how often you contacted something, including your own nose, eyes, or mouth, you'd most likely quit any pretense of checking inside a couple of moments.

As characteristic as it might be, it's through touch that hands become presented to a huge number of hurtful germs and microorganisms every day. Legitimate hand-washing disposes of a large portion of these microorganisms, keeping you and others more advantageous.

Washing your hands appropriately with cleanser and running water can fight off ailments that influence solid individuals just as those with debilitated resistant frameworks.

These sicknesses run from respiratory diseases, for

example, pneumonia to gastric contaminations that cause loose bowels. A large number of these conditions can be deadly to a few, for example, infants and kids. You can pass these germs on, regardless of whether you're not debilitated yourself.

What's the most ideal approach to wash your hands?

Washing your hands with plain cleanser and water has been found to diminish a larger number of microscopic organisms than washing with water alone. Antibacterial cleanser may not be important to utilize each day at home outside of medicinal services settings. Normal cleanser and water can be viable.

Steps for washing hands adequately include:

- Rinse your hands under running water at an agreeable temperature. Warm water isn't more viable than cold water at eliminating germs.
- Apply the sort of cleanser you like best. Cleansers to attempt incorporate fluid equations, froths, and those with creams included.
- Work up foam for a large portion of a moment or

more. Make a point to spread the foam on all pieces of your hands and wrists, including under your fingernails and between your fingers.

- Rinse and dry completely.
- If you're utilizing an open washroom, utilize a paper towel both to kill the spigot and turn the entryway handle while leaving.

When to wash your hands

Visit hand-washing is an individual cleanliness propensity you should utilize each day. Times to wash your hands include:

For nourishment prep and eating

- before, during, and in the wake of planning or preparing nourishment, which is particularly significant on the off chance that you contact crude chicken, eggs, meat or fish
- before eating or drinking

For individual consideration, private exercises, and emergency treatment

- after toileting, both at home or in an open

bathroom

- after changing an infant's diaper or helping a little youngster utilize the latrine
- before changing contact focal points
- after cleaning out your nose or hacking, particularly in case, you're wiped out
- before taking prescriptions, for example, pills or eye drops
- after sexual or cozy action
- before treating a consume or twisted, either on yourself or another person
- after keeping an eye on an individual who is sick

High-traffic puts and messy items

- before and in the wake of using open transportation, particularly on the off chance that you clutch the railings on transports and metros
- after taking care of cash or receipts
- after taking care of family or business trash
- after coming into contact with noticeably messy

surfaces, or when your hands are obviously grimy

Social insurance and different settings

- before and in the wake of treating patients in case you're a clinical expert, for example, a specialist, x-beam professional, or chiropractor

- before and subsequent to treating customers in case you're a cosmetologist, beautician, tattoo craftsman, or aesthetician

- before and subsequent to entering an emergency clinic, specialist's office, nursing home, or other sorts of clinical office

Pet consideration

- after taking care of your pet, particularly on the off chance that they eat crude nourishment

- after strolling your canine or dealing with creature squander

When and how to utilize hand sanitizer

Hand sanitizers are accessible as wipes and in gel structure. They're helpful in a hurried choice to utilize when cleanser and running water aren't promptly accessible.

They shouldn't, nonetheless, be utilized consistently rather than hand-washing, since cleanser and water is increasingly suitable for routinely evacuating soil, flotsam and jetsam, and destructive germs than hand sanitizers.

Utilizing hand sanitizers also much of the time can likewise decrease the quantity of supportive microscopic organisms on all fours.

Take advantage of hand sanitizer by remembering these things:

- Use alcohol based items. It's essential to check fixings and to utilize a sanitizer that contains in any event 60 percent alcohol. Ethanol alcohol and isopropanol alcohol are both worthy sorts.

- Scrub your hands. Utilize the measure of hand sanitizer prescribed on the name and rub it into two hands energetically. Make a point to get all territories of the hands, including the wrists and under nails, similarly as you do when washing.

Rub until they air dry.

- Have some close enough. It's a smart thought to keep some hand sanitizer with you. It can prove to be useful when you walk your canine, travel, or go to class at school.

Hand-washing tips

Keep your skin clean and saturated

Obviously, an overdose of something that is otherwise good can have negative outcomes and this means hand-washing, as well.

Washing your hands continually until they're dry, red, and harsh may imply that you're trying too hard. In the event that your hands become split or drain, they might be progressively inclined to contamination from germs and microscopic organisms.

To maintain a strategic distance from dryness, take a stab at utilizing a saturating cleanser, for example, glycerin, or utilize a hand cream or salve in the wake of washing your hands.

Think about your cleanser and capacity

Since germs can live on ineffectively put away bar cleanser, fluid cleanser might be a superior other option. Fluid cleansers ought to be utilized instead of bar cleansers in schools and in childcare settings.

Try not to go over the edge

In certain individuals, including youngsters, excessively visit hand-washing might be an indication of nervousness or a condition called over the top habitual issue (OCD).

Hand-washing tips for kids

Regardless of whether you're an instructor, guardian, or parent, it very well may be difficult to get children to wash their hands effectively. Here are a few hints and deceives that may help:

- Pick your kid's main tune and make them sing it while washing their hands. On the off chance that it's a short melody, make them sing it twice. They can attempt it once in their own voice and once as a character they love.
- Make up a melody or sonnet that incorporates all the means of good hand-washing and discuss it

with your youngster frequently, particularly in the wake of utilizing the latrine and before suppers.

- Make sure the sink is close enough for little legs and hands, at home and at school.

- Use fun cleansers. These can incorporate froth, a fluid cleanser that changes shading, and those that have kid cordial aromas or brilliantly hued bottles.

- Play a round of thumb war or fingerspell with your kid while hand-washing.

Washing your hands with standard cleanser and running water is an exceptionally successful approach to stop the spread of germs and microorganisms. Hand-washing lessens the danger of respiratory and gastrointestinal infections.

It's essential to wash your hands when dealing with nourishment or eating. Standard, non-antibacterial cleanser is fine for most regular use.

CHAPTER THREE
WHY YOU SHOULD WASH YOUR HANDS

There are an expected 1,500 microorganisms for every square centimeter of skin on your hand. Probably the most ideal approaches to forestall microscopic organisms related ailments and different irresistible ailment is to wash your hands with cleanser and water.

While most everybody has heard this message, examines have indicated that individuals despite everything are not washing their hands the correct way. Truth be told, washing alone isn't sufficient to forestall the spread of microscopic organisms and different germs. In the wake of washing, you should likewise dry your hands completely with a perfect towel or air dryer. Learning great hand-cleanliness propensities is basic to lessening the spread of germs.

Germs Are Everywhere

Germs, for example, microorganisms and infections,

are minuscule and not promptly unmistakable to the unaided eye. Because you can't see them, it doesn't imply that they aren't there. Truth be told, a few microbes live on your skin and some even live inside you. Germs normally dwell on ordinary articles, for example, mobile phones, shopping baskets, and your toothbrush. They can be moved from debased articles to your hands when you contact them. Probably the most well-known ways that germs get moved to your hands are through taking care of crude meat, by utilizing the can, or changing a diaper, by hacking or sniffling, and after contact with pets.

Pathogenic microbes, infections, growths, and different germs cause illness in people. These germs access the body as they are moved from individual to individual or from contact with defiled surfaces. Once inside the body, the germs maintain a strategic distance from the body's safe framework and are equipped for creating poisons that make you wiped out. The most widely recognized reasons for foodborne ailments and food contamination are microorganisms, infections, and parasites. Responses to these germs (a couple of which are recorded beneath) can run from mellow gastric inconvenience and the runs to death.

- MRSA - a sort of superbug, that can cause genuine diseases and are hard to treat because of their protection from anti-infection agents.
- Clostridium difficile - anti-infection safe microorganisms that can cause genuine loose bowels and stomach torment.
- E. coli - pathogenic strains of these microscopic organisms cause intestinal ailment, urinary tract diseases, and meningitis.
- Salmonella - cause the sickness salmonellosis, which brings about queasiness, spewing, stomach torment, and the runs.

How Hand Washing Prevents the Spread of Germs

Appropriate hand washing and drying is the best technique for forestalling the spread of sickness, as it evacuates the earth and germs that can be spread to other people and assists with keeping the earth around you clean. As per the CDC, appropriately washing and drying your hands lessens your danger of becoming ill with the runs by 33 percent. It likewise diminishes your danger of getting a respiratory disease by up to 20 percent.

Having clean hands is significant in light of the fact that individuals frequently utilize their hands to contact their eyes, nose, and mouth. Contact with these territories gives germs, similar to the influenza infection, access to within the body where they can cause disease, and can likewise spread skin and eye contaminations.

You ought to consistently wash your hands in the wake of contacting whatever might be filthy or have a high likelihood of being sullied with germs, for example, crude meat, and subsequent to utilizing the latrine.

Step by step instructions to Wash Your Hands Properly

Washing your hands is a basic procedure that yields incredible medical advantages. The key is by and large sure to wash and dry your hands appropriately to evacuate earth, microorganisms, and different germs.

There are four basic strides to washing your hands. These are:

- Use warm running water to wet your hands while scouring them with cleanser.
- Rub your hands together being certain to foam the rear of the hands and under your nails.
- Scrub your hands completely for in any event 20 seconds.
- Rinse your hands under running water to evacuate the cleanser, soil, and germs.

The Healthiest Way to Dry Your Hands

Drying your hands is a stage that ought not to be overlooked in the cleaning procedure. Appropriately drying your hands does exclude cleaning your hands on your garments to dry them. Drying your hands with a paper towel or utilizing a hand dryer without scouring your hands together is best at keeping microscopic organisms tallies low. Scouring your hands together while drying them under a hand dryer counterbalance the advantages of handwashing by carrying microscopic organisms inside the skin to the surface. These microbes, alongside any that were not expelled by washing, would then be able to be moved to different surfaces.

The most effective method to Use Hand Sanitizers

The best alternative for expelling soil and germs from your hands is cleanser and water. In any case, some hand sanitizers can fill in as an elective when cleanser and water are not accessible. Hand sanitizers ought not to be utilized as a trade for cleanser and water since they are not as compelling at expelling soil or nourishment and oils that may jump on the hands in the wake of eating. Hand sanitizers work by coming into direct contact with microscopic organisms and different germs. The alcohol in the sanitizer separates the bacterial cell film and demolishes the germs. When utilizing a hand sanitizer, be certain that it is alcohol based and contains at any rate 60% alcohol. Utilize a paper towel or fabric to expel any soil or nourishment on your hands. Apply the hand sanitizer as coordinated on the guidelines. Rub the sanitizer all over your hands and between your fingers until your hands are dry.

Hand Sanitizers vs. Soap and Water

Antibacterial hand sanitizers are showcased to general society as a viable method to wash one's hands when customary cleanser and water are not accessible. These "waterless" items are especially famous with guardians of little kids. Makers of hand sanitizers guarantee that the sanitizers execute 99.9 percent of germs. Since you normally use hand sanitizers to purify your hands, the supposition that will be that 99.9 percent of hurtful germs are slaughtered by the sanitizers. Research considers proposing this isn't the situation.

How Do Hand Sanitizers Work?

Hand sanitizers work by stripping ceaselessly the external layer of oil on the skin. This normally forestalls microbes present in the body from rising to the top of the hand. In any case, these microbes that are ordinarily present in the body are commonly not the sorts of microscopic organisms that will make us debilitated. In a survey of the examination, Barbara Almanza, a partner educator at Purdue University who encourages safe sanitation practices to laborers, arrived at a fascinating resolution. She takes note that the examination shows that hand sanitizers don't altogether lessen the number of microorganisms on the hand and now and again may possibly build the measure of microbes. So the inquiry emerges, in what manner can the producers make the 99.9 percent guarantee?

In what capacity can Manufacturers Make the 99.9 Percent Claim?

The makers of the items test the items on microbes corrupted lifeless surfaces; consequently, they can determine the cases of 99.9 percent of microscopic organisms murdered. On the off chance that the items were completely tried on hands, there would no uncertainty be various outcomes. Since there is inalienable intricacy in the human hand, testing hands would be progressively troublesome. Utilizing surfaces with controlled factors is a simpler method to acquire some sort of consistency in the outcomes. Be that as it may, as we are on the whole mindful, regular day to day existence isn't as predictable.

Hand Sanitizer versus Hand Soap and Water

Curiously enough, the Food and Drug Administration, with respect to guidelines concerning legitimate systems for nourishment administrations, prescribes that hand sanitizers not be utilized instead of hand cleanser and water however just as a subordinate. In like manner, Almanza prescribes that to appropriately clean the hands, cleanser, and water ought to be utilized during hand washing. A hand sanitizer cannot and ought not to replace appropriate purifying methods with cleanser and water.

Hand sanitizers can be a valuable elective when the choice of utilizing cleanser and water isn't accessible. A alcohol based sanitizer that contains in any event 60% alcohol ought to be utilized to guarantee that germs are slaughtered. Since hand sanitizers don't evacuate soil and oils on hands, it is ideal to wipe your hands with a towel or napkin before applying the sanitizer.

Shouldn't something be said about Antibacterial Soaps?

Research on the utilization of customer antibacterial cleansers has indicated that plain cleansers are similarly as powerful as antibacterial cleansers in diminishing microscopic organism's related sicknesses. Truth be told, utilizing buyer antibacterial cleanser items may increment bacterial protection from anti-microbials in certain microscopic organisms. These ends just apply to buyer antibacterial cleansers and not to those utilized in medical clinics or other clinical zones. Different investigations propose that ultra-clean situations and the tireless utilization of antibacterial cleansers and hand sanitizers may hinder legitimate invulnerable framework advancement in youngsters. This is on the grounds that provocative frameworks require a more prominent presentation to basic germs for appropriate improvement.

In September 2016, the U.S. Nourishment and Drug Administration restricted the advertising of over-the-counter antibacterial items that contain a few fixings including triclosan and triclocarban. Triclosan in antibacterial cleansers and different items have been connected to the advancement of specific maladies.

Everybody has a type of hand sanitizer in their satchel, around their work area, in the vehicle. Children have hand sanitizers in their book sacks, instructors keep bottles on their work areas and offer wipes to their understudies. In any case, how are successful are these hand sanitizers, particularly the wipes? Are hand purifying wipes powerful?

Despite the fact that the sanitizer creators guarantee that most wipes murder 99.9% of unsafe germs and microorganisms, it is being discovered this isn't generally the situation. Regularly these are tried on lifeless things, not hands, and actually, don't execute that high of a measure of hurtful germs. Quite a bit of what the sterilizing wipes remove isn't even truly what makes individuals wiped out. The best act of just for remaining solid is washing hands in cleanser and water.

In the event that no cleanser and water are accessible than hand sterilizing wipes are better than not cleaning hands by any means, however, they ought not replace hand washing. The sum that hand sanitizers are utilized ought to likewise be kept at any rate, for example, cleanser and water ought to be utilized in the event that it is accessible; on the off chance that it isn't, at that point take out the wipes for use. Some contend that the expanded utilization of hand sterilizing wipes and gels is expanding diseases as they slaughter the great microorganisms expected to battle germs and ailment causing microscopic organisms. Some accept that protections are brought down and ailment is expanded in view of the overutilization of hand sanitizers.

Numerous youngsters are currently acclimated with washing their hands with hand sterilizing items rather than cleanser and water. This is making them not wash their hands adequately when they do utilize cleanser and water as they don't rehearse it enough. Once more, this can prompt expanded ailment.

In any case, there is a spot and time to utilize hand disinfecting wipes. Now and again, it is simply impractical or useful to wash hands with cleanser and water. Maybe a family is in a vehicle and somebody wheezes, utilizes the wipes. Perhaps a sales rep has quite recently warmly greeted a large number of individuals and can't discover cleanser and water, utilize a wipe. Once in a while people don't have the versatility or offices to continually wash hands; this is when wipes can prove to be useful.

Do Hand Sanitizers Really Work to Kill Bacteria?

Hand sanitizer distributors eliminate microscopic

organisms through the dynamic element of alcohol. Alcohol makes up somewhere in the range of 60 to 90 percent of the sanitizer, and anything short of 60 percent may not be compelling in eliminating microscopic organisms. The mystery is the point at which the dynamic element of alcohol is put onto a possibly microscopic organisms filled region, it harms the particles. It will possibly work if the sanitizer is placed into direct contact with the zone tainted.

Hand sanitizer accomplishes take a shot at the hands yet prevents microscopic organisms that might be experienced on surfaces later. It will eliminate microbes on contact, yet it isn't viable after that. This interprets hand sanitizer must be continually utilized, yet the high alcohol substance can dry out the skin and even aggravate it.

Cleanser is altogether different than utilizing a sanitizer. At the point when an individual washes their hands with cleanser, microscopic organisms particles are expelled from the skin. Interestingly, sanitizers simply kill the particles, they are not evacuated. So those particles remain on the skin however never again can bring on any damage. The best procedure is to utilize both, utilizing the sanitizer in the wake of washing hands. Sanitizer ought to be scoured into the hands for roughly thirty seconds, and it truly kills an assortment of microbes. It has been appeared to try and shield from MRSA, a tissue eating microscopic organisms that can be destructive.

To considerably promote the effectively numerous advantages of hand sanitizer, individuals that utilization it likewise show more slow redevelopment of microscopic organisms, everybody has some type of microscopic organisms on their hands at some random time. It doesn't forestall all germs, as some are airborne, yet it is as yet an incredible item.

Despite the fact that hand sanitizer is a great item, it ought not to be utilized for everything, in the event that hands are presented to blood, for instance, they ought to be washed with cleanser and water. Moreover, it isn't acceptable in the nourishment administration industry since hands get wet a great deal from nourishment planning, and doesn't appropriately expel fecal matter on the hands from inappropriate hand washing after bathroom use.

When buying hand sanitizer, check the alcohol content in it. The higher the centralization of alcohol, the more viable it will be. There is even an assortment of fragrances accessible too, and there are even scaled-down allocators that can be placed into a satchel or a movement sack for use too. They ought to be utilized all year, however, they are stunningly better to secure us throughout the winter a long time with numerous infections going around.

CHAPTER FOUR

CAN YOU DRINK HAND SANITIZER OR GET DRUNK ON IT

Chopped You may have caught wind of individuals drinking hand sanitizer to become inebriated or get a buzz. Is it safe? What are the impacts? It's a great opportunity to find the solutions.

Drinking Hand Sanitizer

A commonplace 240 ml compartment of hand sanitizer gel contains about a similar measure of alcohol as five shots of hard alcohol. It's difficult to state when drinking hand sanitizer came into vogue, yet reports of its utilization as an intoxicant with jail detainees began surfacing around 2007. Late patterns, fundamentally rehearsed by adolescents, incorporate blending hand sanitizer with mouthwash to make a solid minty mixed drink, blending the gel in with salt to isolate the alcohol from the gel, and refining the alcohol from hand sanitizer.

Drinking the subsequent mixed drink is designated "hand sanitrippin'," "getting a hand rational soundness fix," "becoming inebriated on Mr. Clean's Tears," or "getting hand sterilized."

Compound Composition of Hand Sanitizer

The issue here is that there are various kinds of alcohol that might be utilized as the disinfectant close by sanitizer and just one of them isn't savage toxic! Methanol isn't utilized close by sanitizer on the grounds that it is poisonous and is assimilated through the skin.

Hand sanitizer containing isopropyl alcohol (scouring alcohol) is utilized close by sanitizer. While it isn't assimilated through the skin as much as methanol, this alcohol is dangerous and will harm your sensory system and interior organs on the off chance that you drink it. Potential impacts may incorporate visual impairment, cerebrum harm, and kidney and liver harm. These impacts might be perpetual. It's likewise conceivable to pass on from drinking this concoction. In spite of the fact that scouring alcohol isn't acceptable to drink, it's improbable an individual would have the option to differentiate the impacts from those brought about by drinking grain alcohol. Drinking isopropyl alcohol at first causes inebriation, slurred discourse obscured vision and tipsiness.

Hand sanitizer containing ethyl alcohol (ethanol or grain alcohol) hypothetically could be tanked, aside from it might be denatured. This implies the alcohol has intentionally been contaminated to make it undrinkable. Back in the times of Prohibition, denaturing operators included arsenic and benzene. Present-day denaturing specialists run from poisonous synthetic compounds to non-dangerous, foul-tasting synthetic concoctions. The issue is that you can't tell from the name which denaturing compound was utilized.

Hand Sanitizer Ingredient List

At the point when you read a jug of hand sanitizer, you'll likely observe ethyl alcohol recorded as the dynamic fixing, around 60% to 95%. This is identical to 120-proof alcohol. In correlation, straight vodka is just 80-proof. Other (idle) fixings incorporate benzophenone-4, carbomer, aroma, glycerin, isopropyl myristate, propylene glycol, tocopheryl acetic acid derivation, and water. A portion of these fixings are innocuous, while others are poisonous. Of this example list, the aroma is the added substance destined to cause issues. You can't tell the creation of the aroma and numerous normal aromas are gotten from petrochemicals.

Would you be able to Drink It?

You can drink hand sanitizer, yet basically you shouldn't. Regardless of whether the mark records ethyl alcohol as the main dynamic fixing, it's improbable that alcohol is in a drinkable structure. Additionally, different fixings might be harmful. Truly, it's conceivable to distill alcohol from hand sanitizer, yet you'll likely have a low-immaculateness (polluted) item.

The fundamental danger of drinking hand sanitizer isn't from the harmful synthetic concoctions yet from the incredibly high alcohol content. The vast majority who are hospitalized from drinking hand sanitizer is there in view of alcohol harming (a alcohol overdose). The alcohol content is high to the point that it is anything but difficult to drink a perilous measure of alcohol before feeling the underlying impacts.

- There are various definitions of hand sanitizer, yet every one of them incorporates synthetic concoctions that make drinking it hazardous.

- It is conceivable to get inebriated by drinking hand sanitizer made utilizing ethyl alcohol or ethanol.

- Other kinds of alcohol might be utilized as a disinfectant close by sanitizer, including isopropyl alcohol or scouring alcohol. Isopropyl Alcohol is harmful.

- Even if an item is liberated from denaturing specialists, scents, or different added substances, drinking hand sanitizer is hazardous in light of the fact that it contains higher percent alcohol than mixed refreshment. There is an extraordinary danger of alcohol harming or overdose.

- It's conceivable to distill ethanol from hand sanitizer to cleanse it. The refined item will at present contain some degree of debasement.

Hand Washing and Hand Sanitizers - Handy

Advice on How to Prevent the Spread of Germs

You might be astonished to discover that 80% of all contaminations are transmitted by hands. I realize I was the point at which I heard this measurement. That is the awful news. The uplifting news? Basic great cleanliness can forestall the spread of germs and the transmission of microscopic organisms and infections that can cause sickness. This is particularly significant during cold and influenza season and unique occasions, which are the most significant seasons to ward germs off. All things considered, who needs to become ill during these unique occasions?

This is what you have to know. Fundamentally, there are two decisions.

First on the rundown is antiquated hand washing. You have to wash your hands in the best possible way and regularly. Hand washing 101: Wet your hands with warm, running water, apply cleanser, at that point foam, and make certain to rub them energetically with a cleanser for at least 15 seconds. It's critical to clean between your fingers, under your fingernails, the backs of your hands and even your wrists. You should wash your hands well and dry them with a perfect towel or paper towel. Here's a tip: utilize a paper towel to kill the fixtures and open the entryway when you exit, as they are both germ bearers.

When to wash your hands? You would figure it would be an easy decision, yet clearly there are many individuals out there who don't wash when they should. Here are a few instances of when you have to wash your hands: when getting ready nourishment, before eating, in the wake of sniffling or hacking, cleaning out your nose, utilizing an open washroom, taking care of pets, evolving diapers, doing the clothing, utilizing your remote control, PC console, etc.

Hand washing is easy to do and powerful in forestalling the spread of germs.

Having said that, life is occupied and access to cleanser and water isn't constantly conceivable. A choice to hand washing is utilizing a hand sanitizer. There are alcohol and non-alcohol hand sanitizers. Both adequately kill 99.9% of germs inside 15 seconds, yet non-alcohol hand sanitizers are delicate, non-dangerous, non-combustible and safe for your entire family.

Alcohol based sanitizers dry your skin, making little splits and hole - immaculate concealing spots for frightful malady causing microscopic organisms!

A alcohol-free hand sanitizer contains germ-murdering Benzalkonium Chloride, and it feels preferred on your skin over alcohol based sanitizers. It leaves no clingy buildup and leaves your skin delicate, saturated and, in particular, germ-free. Also, a hand sanitizer is compelling in eliminating germs that can cause sickness, including the Norwalk Virus, SARS, Avian Flu, Salmonella, E. coli, and that's only the tip of the iceberg.

Another beneficial thing about hand sanitizers is that you can take them with you when you're all over the place, when hand washing may not be conceivable. Many come in smaller than normal showers that advantageously fit into your pocket, wallet, handbag, knapsack, PC pack or folder case. Some offer huge sizes for your home that your entire family can utilize. Also, in case you're going for business or delight, the smaller than usual showers make great mates. You can take them with you whether you're touring or unwinding in the sun on lovely seashore.

Utilizing a hand sanitizer is basic. Simply apply a thumbnail add up to your palm, simply enough so your skin feels wet. Rub it into your hands until dry. Inside 15 seconds it will have killed 99.9% of sickness causing germs.

The fundamental objective is to remain healthy, and both handwashing and hand sanitizers give superb alternatives to forestalling the spread of ailment causing germs. Anticipation is precious.

A great many people have presumably heard at once or another that hand sanitizer is viable in eliminating germs. Truly, this is valid; however for what reason is it so powerful? Is it better to wash your hands with cleanser and water or utilize a hand purifying item? These are a portion of the inquiries that were irritating me, so I did a little research.

Hand sanitizers work due to their high centralizations of alcohol, and alcohol murders most germs and microscopic organisms. On the off chance that you rub alcohol on your hands for around 30 seconds, it will kill numerous types of microscopic organisms and infections. An intriguing measurement to note is that an individual who utilizes sanitizer is likewise prone to show a slower redevelopment of microscopic organisms. Everybody has a few microbes on their hands consistently, yet hand sanitizers eases back the development of microscopic organisms whenever utilized appropriately.

It has been demonstrated that the utilization of hand sanitizers and different types of handwashing in schools significantly lessens ailment rates and results in better participation records. Alcohol based sanitizer can likewise be more compelling than hand washing sometimes in light of the fact that it's is simpler and snappier to utilize. All together for handwashing to be really powerful, you should utilize warm water, cleanser, and foam for around 2 minutes. A great many people are excessively restless for this, so hand washing isn't totally compelling in murdering the microscopic organisms on your hands. Hand sanitizers, then again, can be conveyed with you in little containers and take just around 30 seconds to eliminate germs.

Everybody should realize that while hand sanitizers are incredible much of the time, they are not the best decision for ALL cleaning needs. Hand sanitizer isn't powerful in the nourishment administration industry where hands are much of the time wet during readiness. Hand sanitizer doesn't evacuate fecal make a difference on hands after poor hand-washing following washroom use. What's more, having contact with earth or organic liquids requires energetic hand washing. Hand sanitizers ought not to supplant handwashing in all occurrences, yet it very well may be an extraordinary method to eliminate germs and microscopic organisms, particularly when you're in a hurry.

CHAPTER FIVE
HEALTH AND HAND SANITATION

One of our significant worries in our wellbeing and keeping us bereft of germs and bacterial contamination is with the assistance of hand sanitizer distributors. With all the destructive ailments and pandemics that we have experienced previously, it is significant for us to remain ensured and keep up the neatness of ourselves and our environmental factors on what our eyes can see, however even those that we can't.

In our day by day lives, we ought to know about where the most tainting and spread of infection is conceivable. Swarmed and much of the time visited places like tram stations and other open vehicles are wellsprings of the microscopic organisms that you may even bring home. It is then imperative to have a convenient hand sanitizer allocator in your pack when voyaging. On the off chance that you have the opportunity to wash your hands when you go to a solace room, do as such. This ought to likewise help in shielding yourself from microscopic organisms that you may get. On the off chance that a hand sanitizer is accessible in a similar restroom, profit yourself of the benefit.

Every now and again passed on things like bills and coins have been passed around may bring infections. That shopping basket that you've been pushing around the grocery store, the entryway in the cafe or the counter in the bank may all have been taken care of by such a significant number of individuals that you can't tell which even got you contaminated. It is then essential to shield yourself from being moved to you by disinfecting your hands after each taking care of.

There have been hand sanitizer gadgets, particularly those divider mounted in various open zones like grocery stores, cafés, and trams. You may as often as possible disregard this propensity for disinfecting however when you do see a hand sanitizer container in any of these territories, take the risk and shield yourself from conceivable wellbeing concerns. Besides helping yourself and your friends and family, you can likewise secure people around you with infections that you yourself may not realize you have.

Subsequent to washing your hands in the washroom, there are cleanser and hand sanitizer allocators accessible for you. In spite of the fact that washing your hands may expel noticeable soil and smell, there are those which you can't see. Hand sanitizers are a decent method for guaranteeing that 99.9 percent of the germs that you collected is disposed of. At the point when you are in the eatery, there are additionally hand sanitizer gadgets on their counters. Get a couple of drops onto your hands before eating to ensure you are not ruining your feast with microorganisms.

Any place you might be, regardless of whether at home or grinding away or even while in a hurry it is critical to be cautious about what we uncover ourselves with. At the point when you are outside the house, you are inclined to various conceivable disease-causing microscopic organisms. So when you return home, there are odds of taking them home as well. Aside from a decent cleanliness, purify yourself and your friends and family at home. Have hand sanitizer distributors in the kitchen and in the washrooms for a solid, straightforward and without germ living.

For what reason Does Hand Sanitizer Kill Germs?

Hand sanitizer is another purifying item that is rapidly assuming control over the capacity of cleanser and water. It has solid disinfectant properties and contains liquor, which can maybe eliminate germs more successfully than the old strategy for washing your hands. Sanitizer comes in froth, fluid, or gel and is made by various organizations in a wide range of size containers.

It is a moderately new item that is gigantically helpful. Numerous individuals convey little containers in their satchels or pockets to help watch them against germs when they don't approach sinks. Some have gotten over the top about it, utilizing it on their hands at whatever point they open an entryway or contact any bit of product.

Businesses likewise love it and appropriate free sanitizer to their representatives. A few organizations necessitate that everybody wash their hands with it in the wake of contacting the entryway handles or time clock. This helps hold disorder in line and shields more individuals from taking days off. Creation would then be able to remain consistent all during the influenza season. This is frequently a major issue, particularly for individuals who work near one another in workplaces and need to share telephones, PCs, and gear.

Sanitizers accompany certain marks of shame and difficulties, however. There are a couple of gatherings who are drastically against utilizing them. Two fundamental reasons are the reason for any turmoil. The primary explanation is that numerous individuals figure cleanser and high temp water can carry out the responsibility fine and dandy, if worse. It, now and again, improves - yet this is on the grounds that numerous individuals frequently don't utilize sanitizer effectively.

A few people put only a smidgen on all fours their palms together. This doesn't do especially for your hand all in all, germs despite everything life. Individuals contend for water and cleanser since it powers your whole hands to get spotless and the hotness of the water can eliminate germs well. What you should accomplish for the sanitizer is to put a ton on all fours rub it all over - in the middle of your fingers, on the rear of your hands, in any event, getting it around your fingernails as much as you can.

There is another enemy of sanitizer battle with respect to it being excessively powerful at eliminating germs. Most murder precisely what they publicize they slaughter: 99.9 percent of microorganisms. Yet, this can be shockingly hindering to your wellbeing. Individuals need a modest quantity of microorganisms all together for their invulnerable framework to watch appropriately against it. In the event that you abandon certain microscopi from it and have gotten more grounded. There has c organisms for significant stretches of time; it can make you extremely wiped out when you at last experience it once more.

You additionally need to stress over the .01 percent of germs that remaining parts alive after you attempted to murder it, it may not appear as though they can do a lot, yet by enduring the counter bacterial cleanser, they have constructed a protection been an incredible media dread about making super-microorganisms which are practically difficult to slaughter. The best activity, along these lines, isn't to mishandle sanitizer. Utilize high temp water and cleanser at whatever point you can and use sanitizer just for awkward occasions.

You can even appreciate the advantages of mix sanitizers and creams. Many bodies and magnificence organizations have understood that there isn't a point in making sanitizers and salves independent. By consolidating them, you can be perfect and work on making smooth skin simultaneously.

Which Hand Sanitizer is Right for You?

Have you at any point needed a hand cleaner however you're not near a washroom and aren't outfitted with hand cleanser? For an in a hurry, occupied way of life, hand sanitizer is an incredible method to avoid germs and keep your hands clean. While a few people might know that hand sanitizers are compelling for eliminating germs without water, many may not think about the various brands and structures that liquor sanitizers come in. I might want to layout for both of you of the main brands and a portion of their advantages and confinements.

Purell

The entirety of Purell's hand cleanliness items arrive in a hand gel recipe. The most straightforward approach to buy Purell hand gel is in an 8 oz. siphon bottle. Purell has 5 fundamental items that they produce and sell. They are Purell moment hand sanitizer, Purell with aloe, Purell dampness treatment, Purell spring sprout, and Purell sea fog. Purell is a notable brand whose items can be found in most medications and supermarkets. While mass size jugs are genuinely cheap peruse, the movement size containers can get entirely expensive.

Germ X

Germ X offers an assortment of hand disinfecting items that arrive in a variety of sizes. They go from 1 oz. as far as possible up to 40 oz. They have unique hand sanitizer, Germ X with aloe, just as a few scented hand sanitizers. They have likewise as of late built up a lavender hand disinfecting splash, and a no-mess hand purifying froth. You can discover numerous Germ X items at your nearby medication or market; nonetheless, you are probably going to just observe their most fundamental items on the racks. Their increasingly particular items, for example, the hand purifying shower or froth will be progressively hard to find.

While hand sanitizer gels appear to be the most widely recognized structure, they will, in general, be the least attractive because of the time span it takes to assimilate into your skin and dry totally. With all hand sanitizers, it is critical to ensure they have a cream included or the liquor can negatively affect your skin.

CHAPTER SIX
HOW DOES HAND SANITIZER WORK

You have likely heard that hand sanitizers are successful hand cleaners that eliminate germs and microorganisms, yet have you at any point considered how a straightforward liquor based hand sanitizer could be as powerful as washing completely with hand cleanser and water? Hand cleanser and water lift the germs off our skin and flush them away while hand sanitizers simply slaughter the germs on contact. This is really exceptional, and the inquiry is how?

Hand sanitizers are comprised of ethyl liquor, idle added substances, for example, water, different alcohols, and aromas. Ethyl liquor is the dynamic fixing and is intended to eliminate germs. Something imperative to think about ethyl liquor is that it's just successful if the centralization of liquor is somewhere in the range of 60 and 95%. Any under 60% won't be sufficiently adequate to eliminate germs and is trivial in utilizing. Numerous specialists prompted that it's imperative to take a gander at the marks close by sanitizers to ensure that you're getting a quality item with adequate groupings of liquor.

There are two general kinds of scouring liquor: ethyl liquor and isopropyl liquor. The two sorts eliminate microscopic organisms adequately yet are not as compelling on infections. As the liquor dissipates, it sucks out the inner parts of microorganisms and infections and murders them. Be that as it may, the microbes or infections won't be dead until all the liquor has vanished. One thing to note is that isopropyl liquor requires around 10 minutes on the skin's surface to eliminate microscopic organisms, giving ethyl liquor and favorable position over isopropyl liquor.

At the point when you apply the hand sanitizer, make certain to rub all aspects of the skin on your hands completely in light of the fact that this is what's going to murder the germs. Hand sanitizers won't get past natural liquids, soil, blood or other grime to eliminate germs. These things must be washed away before a hand sanitizer is applied. Additionally, the liquor close by sanitizer has a drying impact, so it's a smart thought to utilize some kind of hand or body cream in the wake of utilizing hand sanitizer.

Battle Germs with Purell Instant Hand Sanitizer

Today it is a higher priority than at any other time to battle germs with Purell Instant Hand Sanitizer. Clinical science makes a valid statement in saying that keeping hands clean and germ-free is perhaps the best advance to avert germs and infections. Since hands go all over the place, they are generally well-suited to get germs en route. Contacting shared phones, PC consoles, door handles, and remote gadgets are the most regular approach to get and transmit live germs from articles to the body. Before the individual knows it, they have gotten a germ from a surface, put it into their mouth, and tainted themselves with colds, infections, and hazardous sicknesses, for example, the H1N1 Swine Flu.

Gojo Industries is a main producer of items for cleaning, and their Purell Instant Hand Sanitizer is perhaps the most recent expansion to their line of germ battling items. Purell Hand Sanitizer is utilized in light of the fact that it works so well, in broad daylight places, stores, cafés and different spots where you might not approach cleanser and water. It is a significant item to have accessible at kid daycare focuses, schools, libraries, and different structures frequented by youths and children for that additional measure of assurance and neatness.

Give a first line of safeguard at your home or office with Purell Hand Sanitizer. Buy in mechanical sizes, little work area gadgets, or divider units. Different sizes and sorts of containers are accessible for kitchens, restrooms, and other regular zones. It's an ounce of anticipation that can venture to spare lives, and absolutely cut down on infection and ailments.

Purell Hand Sanitizer kills 99.9% of germs in around 15 seconds. It bodes well to have Purell Sanitizers helpful for all to use around the working environment or out in the open spots. It is dermatologist tried and leaves hands feeling delicate and saturated even with visit use. Purell Hand Sanitizer is accessible in fluid-structure and moist disposable clothes for additional accommodation.

Utilizing germ battling items in the work environment is an extraordinary method to diminish debilitated time because of ailment and to help forestall the spread of influenza, colds, and different illnesses among collaborators. Use busy working and at home, with a few allocators put around inside the structures. Emergency clinics, centers, schools, and open structures need to give germ care items on account of their size. Any association or business that draws huge hordes of individuals to their site ought to have Purell Hand Sanitizer accessible for advantageous use to stop the spread of germs.

Fantasies Regarding Hand Sanitizer Dispensers

There isn't a day that passes by that you don't come into contact with germs and unsafe microscopic organisms. Germs are all over the place, so germs winding up on you are inescapable. Visit contact on normal, ordinary things enables germs to spread. Door handles, PC consoles, and level surfaces are only a couple of the most mainstream places germs can be found. In any case, what would you be able to do to assist battle with offing hurtful microbes and germs? Many have gone to hand sanitizers. Hand sanitizers are an incredible answer to assist you with battling of germs. Anyway, there are several fantasies flowing about these distributors that are positively false. These incorporate the accompanying.

Fantasy

All hand sanitizer containers are the equivalent

This is bogus. Indeed there are many sorts of containers available. The best gadgets are those that you don't need to come into contact with so as to get the hand sanitizer. The way to maintaining a strategic distance from germs is to just not contact anything you don't need to. Regardless of whether you're utilizing an open bathroom and exploiting contact-free bathroom advancements, or essentially utilizing an independent hand sanitizer allocator, not contacting hardware can decrease the danger of coming into contact with germs.

Past the hand's free gadgets, many expect you to pick the gel or the froth. Some select distributors really give you the alternatives about what you might want to see administered. These are the decision by a developing number of associations. You ought to likewise be watching out for those that are dribble safe and meet CDC, APIC and OSHA benchmarks. These sorts of containers are the most noteworthy of value and meet each sanitation need.

Hand sanitizer distributors make tranquilize safe freak microscopic organisms

This is bogus. Basically, liquor, being the principle fixing close by sanitizer distributors, eliminates germs. There has been no proof that bolsters the hypothesis that germs change to supplant the impacts of hand sanitizer. Actually, liquor based hand sanitizers have been appeared to execute even multi-medicate safe pathogens

Legends are only that - fantasies. The most ideal approach to know for certain if a container is the best possible cleanliness answer for you is to just do a little research. There is a colossal measure of research and science that goes into the cosmetics of hand sanitizer. The objective is to help secure you by murdering the germs you can without much of a stretch come into contact with consistently. Know about your environment and put forth a traditionalist attempt to just touch things in broad daylight places you need to contact. It is additionally imperative to recall that you should wash your hands oftentimes for the duration of the day and to abstain from contacting your eyes, nose or mouth during the day.

Laws of Hand Sanitizers

Everybody should know at this point hand sanitizer is basic for keeping up wellbeing and keeping your safe framework shielded from germs. The Centers for Disease Control (CDC) have educated us that notwithstanding washing your hands every now and again and completely, utilizing a hand sanitizer to wipe out germs is exceptionally useful in lessening your hazard for colds and flus, among different sicknesses. Here are the 3 Laws to search for when searching out a decent hand sanitizer.

The Law of Effectiveness

So as to be feasible as a disinfecting item, you need a hand sanitizer that WORKS. There are numerous items available, yet the FDA has explicitly affirmed certain substances as antimicrobial operators. One of those substances is ethyl liquor. In the right sums, ethyl liquor can be 99.9% powerful against germs. The normal sum is between 62-70% by volume. On the off chance that a hand sanitizer doesn't contain an FDA-endorsed tranquilize like ethyl liquor, you can't be sure that it is compelling.

The Law of Application

Hand purifying isn't something that most of individuals do all the time. The issue is that they should, however, most hand sanitizers are an agony to apply. You need to pull out a small jug, pop the top, press the gel out in the perfect sum, and attempt to spread it around on your hands before it slides off or dissipates. For individuals with multiple hands that is a basic accomplishment, however, for all of us, it's somewhat entangled. The best hand sanitizer application is through a shower bottle, which gives you the perfect sum per splash and is extremely easy to do with two hands. In the event that you can't make a difference the hand sanitizer effectively, for what reason would you be roused to utilize it?

The Law of Moisture

Liquor is a dissolvable that extricates characteristic oils from things it contacts, including your skin. At the point when your skin loses its regular oils, it dries out. This can be agonizing but ANOTHER motivation behind why individuals would prefer not to utilize hand sanitizers. That is the reason the Law of Moisture says get a hand sanitizer with aloe or a fundamental oils! The liquor will vanish after you've scoured it around to eliminate germs and afterward you'll be left with a charming saturating arrangement that will shield your hands from getting split and sore.

Adhere to these laws and you will locate an extraordinary hand-disinfecting item that won't be an agony to utilize! Hand disinfecting is probably the most ideal approaches to abstain from becoming ill, so don't be apprehensive any longer - keep the 3 Laws of Hand Sanitizers and ensure yourself!

CONCLUSION

In conclusion, most hand sanitizers, with the exception of the "green" assortment, are liquor based. This is on the grounds that liquor eliminates germs viably, and there has been no investigation that demonstrates than anything can demolish germs and microscopic organisms in a hand sterilizing item superior to liquor. The Mayo Clinic even cautions us that a significant number of these new "earth cordial" purging items don't, in reality, clean and eliminate germs as successfully as those that are liquor based. During a time when infections appear to flourish, visit hand washing and the utilization of compelling sanitizers is an unquestionable requirement.

There are the individuals who guarantee that the liquor fixing in most hand sanitizers can hurt our skin and that is consistent with a specific degree. A lot of utilization of liquor based items will in general dry the skin of our hands - however, we can generally utilize a salve to try to shield our hands from looking and feeling dry. It is likewise fitting to ensure that we utilize a sanitizer for our hands yet in addition to things that we routinely use and contact, for example, a console, phone, purses, and even our PDAs.

As indicated by an ongoing Fox News study, there are more microbes present on the base of our sacks than that on our latrine seat. Actually, e-coli and different sorts of microscopic organisms have been found on the base of our totes due to the propensity for putting them down basically anyplace - even on the floors of open restrooms.

www.ingramcontent.com/pod-product-compliance
Lightning Source LLC
Chambersburg PA
CBHW070300220526
45465CB00004B/1677